The Science of Self Massage

Independently Relieve Stress Using Techniques That Target Trigger Points

By K.W. Williams

Table of Contents

Introduction

There is nothing more delightful than visiting a masseuse and having your stress, tension, muscle aches, and old sports injuries kneaded out. But sometimes it is difficult to afford the one hundred dollar an hour or more fees that professional massage therapists charge. You may also not know of a good massage therapist that you can trust with your body. Massage is, after all, a very intimate and even painful experience and you need someone who knows what he or she is doing. Perhaps you have a massage appointment coming up, but you need some quick relief now. For these reasons, it's important that you learn the art of self-massaging.

Self-massaging is an affordable and helpful way for you to give yourself the relief that your sore muscles need. But it is quite important that you learn how to perform self-massaging the correct way to prevent injury to yourself. Just vigorously rubbing your shoulder knots may only make your pain worse in the end. Rolling your feet a little too hard on tennis balls can also cause more harm than good. This book explores some techniques that can help you really improve your self-massaging methods and the level of relief you receive from self-massaging.

Self-massaging is great for muscle pain and recovering from injuries. It can also help you ease emotional issues, since many emotional problems and stresses manifest in the body in the form of physical aches and pains. You can relieve stomach issues and other internal organ problems by targeting specific acupressure points that relate to said internal organ. Basically, self-massaging allows you to treat all of your ailments with some targeted rubbing or pressure application. You can even use heat or cold to help provide yourself relief.

In this book, you will learn about using acupressure and acupuncture methods on yourself in a safe way. You will also learn easy, quick massages that you can perform on yourself at work, in the car, or walking around the grocery store with minimal effort. You will learn about major and minor ailments that you can quickly treat with a little massage. Finally, you will learn about how to spread the love to your loved ones, by becoming the family masseuse.

This book is far from a professional guide. Rather, it is a simple guide for the layperson to use to learn basic massage techniques. If you want to learn more, continue your massage journey with research. There is always more to learn in this complex and wonderful art. The more you know and the more you practice, the better you become.

Chapter 1: The Secrets of Massage

Rules

To perform a massage without injuring yourself or others, you must learn some rules. These rules are meant to protect you from injuring yourself. Failure to follow these rules can result in your injury.

You should always consult a doctor before you attempt a massage on yourself if you suffer from an injury or any type of illness. Never massage yourself to relieve any kind of injury or illness if your doctor advises against it. Doctors tend to err on the side of caution and you do know your body best, but you should try to always to follow your doctor's advice.

When it comes to massaging others, you need to be extremely careful to avoid hurting the person. Don't press down too hard; in fact, it is better to start out by being too gentle, and only increase the pressure you use if your subject requests it. Also don't bend or stretch the individual that you are massaging. Have him or her perform stretches before the massage begins.

Never perform a foot massage or full body massage on a pregnant woman. If you are pregnant yourself, you should also be very careful when self-massaging. A lot of pregnant women suffer from back pain and sore feet, so they crave massage, but unfortunately hitting certain pressure spots can effectively send a pregnant woman into labor. Performing any kind of massage is actually a very dangerous thing to do on a pregnant woman. Speak with a doctor before you attempt any kind of self-massaging if you're pregnant or before you perform a massage on a pregnant woman. A massage professional can be used to help induce labor through massage, but one must exercise extreme caution when doing this. There are certain types of pregnancy massages that are safe for pregnant women because they do not trigger labor, but it is best to leave these massages to professionals. Do not attempt them on your own.

It is best to never eat or work out before a massage. At least wait an hour before you begin a massage after eating or exercising. Waiting longer is even better. You don't have to fast all day to perform a massage and you don't have to postpone a much-needed tension headache rub because you just ate, but eating or working out before a massage can cause greater discomfort.

Massage is not supposed to hurt. Yes, it may feel uncomfortable, but there should be a level of pleasure or release with the discomfort. If something hurts a lot when you rub it, you should stop. Sensitive, tender areas can be revisited later and worked on over time, but don't keep attacking an area that hurts during the same massage. Keep in mind that you don't have to torture yourself to get results. Often, gentle, delicate pressure is sufficient for results, even if it doesn't seem like it. Just pressing down slightly on an acupressure trigger point or a sore muscle often will do a lot more than you realize. If you are hurting or bruising yourself, you are using too much force, and you can ease up and still experience successful results.

Using instruments for massage, such as rollers, tennis balls, or other objects, can be helpful. But you must take care not to apply too much force. It is easier to cause injury with an instrument than with your own hands. Always stop if you start to hurt yourself, or if your subject complains of being hurt.

When you perform a massage, either on yourself or others, you need to have clean hands. You also need to wash your hands following the massage. Why? There are two good reasons. One, you don't want to introduce oils and bacteria from your hands to the pores in the skin on the body, as this can lead to acne and infections. The friction from massage can open these pores, making them more susceptible to these oils and bacteria.

Also, the human body is full of energy. As you will learn in the section on acupressure, this energy flows through the body in what is known as meridians. Often, when you have tight muscles or knots, this is where energy becomes caught up. The blockage in energy can disrupt the health and harmony of the overall body, leading to various health issues and muscle pains. When you massage yourself or someone else, you are using pressure to break up these blockages and hence you absorb a lot of stagnant and even negative energy. This energy can build up in your hands, and can disrupt your energy further. Washing your hands cleanses this energy away and helps you get rid of it for good.

Massage is meant to be relaxing.

Therefore, you may find that a massage makes you very sleepy or drowsy. Be careful when you do a massage before you need to perform a task that requires your wakefulness, such as driving. You don't want to fall asleep while in rush hour on your commute home. It is often best to perform self-massaging before bed, or when you have quiet time to relax at home or in some other safe space.

You can certainly utilize the help of others in receiving a massage. But make sure that other people understand and follow these rules. Be verbal and let them know if they are hurting you when they use too much pressure, for instance. Make sure that they always wash their hands before and after the massage. It is best to not let people walk on your back or pop your back, as this actually can contribute to worsening posture and spinal problems. If you need your spine straightened or a serious muscle injury worked on, consider going to a professional instead of using the help of family or friends. You want someone who really knows how to help you to work on you.

Keep in mind that everyone's bodies are different. What works for one person may not work for another. You may find that certain massages don't feel good to you or that certain techniques don't work for you. You may find that you need more pressure or more voltage from a tens unit or violet wand than most people, or you may find the opposite is true. You may even find that certain rules don't seem to apply to you; for instance, you may prefer cold therapy when most people tell you to use hot. You know yourself best, so do what feels right to you. As long as you are not hurting yourself, you have wiggle room to adapt self-massaging to your unique needs.

Don't expect to cure yourself of a chronic health problem or pain overnight. One massage by a professional is often insufficient to cure you of an issue for life; you need many consecutive treatments over time. It is the same with self-massaging. You will need to work on yourself over time to see any results. Often, you may need to visit a professional to cure chronic back issues, for instance. It is easy to think that massage will solve all of your problems, and indeed massage is a great step toward recovery and wellness, but it will not cure you immediately. It takes time and work.

Finally, it is best to always use a lotion or massage oil. If you don't, you can give yourself a form of rug burn by rubbing your skin with your hands for too long. Your hands tend to be much rougher than the skin on your body, leading to very uncomfortable and unpleasant friction. Lotion is acceptable, but most drugstore lotions do not provide enough lubrication to prevent the irritating friction that rubbing your skin or someone else's skin can bring about. Be sure to keep applying lotion to your hands as soon as your hands start to feel rough. There are expensive and fancy massage oils available on the market that can be great to use, but you don't have to spend lots of money for a good oil. The best oils for massage are actually natural vegetable, nut, or plant oils that you can purchase at your local health food store. Almond, grapeseed, olive, argan, coconut, sunflower, sesame, and safflower oils are all great options that usually only cost a few dollars per bottle. You can also try a shea butter or coconut butter. These oils are great for your skin and usually won't clog your pores, causing infections and acne. If you can buy organic, that is even better, as organic oils and butters tend to have fewer chemicals residues from pesticides and fertilizers to contaminate your body. Store your massage oil in a room temperature, dark place and keep it covered or bottled in order to keep out impurities like dirt and flies. I advise against using unnatural or synthetic products, such as petroleum jelly or baby oil. These products tend to stick and also irritate sensitive skin, leading to breakouts and irritated hair follicles.

You can even make your own massage oil, if you so choose. Use a scented essential oil for seduction, relaxation, or whatever other effect you desire. Mix it with a vegetable or nut oil, or a lotion. The oils will separate, so be sure to shake and stir the emulsion before using it for massage.

Kinds of Massage

There are many different kinds of massage that come from different cultures. What is interesting is that almost all cultures have some form of massage, indicating how important massage is for health and comfort to human beings universally. You can learn the techniques of many different cultures, and incorporate them into your practice.

Abhyanga

Abhyanga is a very unique form of Ayurvedic massage that comes from India. In this form of massage, you use warm oil to release the tension that your muscles hold onto. Never use oil that is hot enough to burn your skin. The benefits of Abhyanga are innumerable. They include replenishing your energy, restoring your skin, stopping the signs of aging, increasing your flexibility, improving your circulation, lubricating your joints, cleansing your body of impurities and toxins, and moving your lymph flow to increase your immune system's power. Wow, right?

It is recommended that you rub warm oil onto your body for fifteen to twenty minutes. All you need is a fourth cup of oil, warmed in a coffee mug in the microwave or in a sauce pan over the stove. Test the oil on your inner wrist to ensure that it is not unbearably hot. In a comfortable room, strip down and dip your hands into the oil, gathering a conservative amount in your palms. The goal is to gently lubricate your skin, not drench yourself and run out of warm oil before the massage is over. Always begin by rubbing the oil into your face in circular motions. Then rub it onto your arms in long, smooth strokes. Move your hands in circles over your knees and elbows. Also rub your belly and chest with large circular strokes. You do not have to get your back or buttocks, but you can if you can reach these areas with ease. Finally, sweep down the legs and spend a few minutes focusing on rubbing the oil into your feet in circular motions. The sweeping and circular motions are meant to stimulate your energy, while the oil is meant to provide lubrication and heighten your body's vibrational energy in tune with the energy of the plant or nut that the oil is made from.

Conclude this massage with a nice warm bath or shower. Pat your body dry with a towel afterward; don't vigorously rub yourself dry. You want to relax totally and release stress and impurities by moving very gently.

Now, Ayurvedic medicine stresses that each person is unique and requires different things. This system of medicine splits people into three main physical groups called doshas: Pitta, Vata, and Kapha. A healthy person is a balance of all three doshas, while an unhealthy person tends to have the traits of mostly one dosha and therefore is predisposed to that dosha's health issues. It is possible to have various traits from more than one dosha, which is what makes Ayurveda complicated. When it comes to Abhyanga, the kind of oil you use depends on which dosha your body falls into. Determining what dosha you are in depends on a lot of factors that fall beyond the scope of this book. However, here are some basic rules that can help you estimate which dosha you belong in so that you can determine what oil you need to use to balance yourself out while using Abhyanga. To form a more accurate image of which group you fall into, you can perform more research on Ayurvedic doshas and even take tests online. Generally, Pittas are often thin, with cold feet and hands, dry or itchy skin, brittle or dry hair, and a tendency toward insomnia and nervousness. Often, they are cold and they prefer to stay in warm environments. Vattas are usually medium or average weight with normal appetites, have reddish skin that is prone to irritation, and have irritable natures too. Their hair is usually healthy and they have flexible joints, and they tend to be hot most of the time. They find it easy to sleep. Kaphas have waxy or oily skin, dark hair, dark eyes, and a tendency to be overweight. They are usually easygoing people who prefer to play supporting roles in others' lives. They have difficulties waking up in the morning and tend to oversleep.

If you are Pitta, you should use coconut or sunflower oil in your massage. Vattas should use sesame or almond. Kaphas should use safflower. All three types of people can use jojoba oil. You can also look up Ayurvedic medicine sites and order massage oils or essential oils created specifically for balancing energy for Vattas, Pittas, or Kaphas.

Acupuncture

Acupuncture is the art of piercing the skin at certain key spots to improve energy flow throughout the body and stimulate the skin. I cover this in more depth in Chapter 3.

Acupressure

Acupressure is the art of stimulating certain spots on the body to regulate energy flow. It is Chinese in origin. I cover acupressure in depth in Chapter 3. Acupressure is a cornerstone of self-massaging therapy because it is relatively easy to apply to yourself.

Swedish Massage

Swedish massage is perhaps the most common and popular form of massage in America. You have probably receive a Swedish massage if you have visited a spa or traditional massage therapist. Swedish massage is often what is depicted in movies and TV shows. This form of massage involves working all the muscles of the body for deep relaxation.

Performing Swedish massage on yourself is often difficult, since you cannot reach every muscle of your body on your own. However, you can still use the techniques of Swedish massage on yourself in small ways. Using a Swedish technique known as Tapotement. Using both your fingertips and the side of your hand, you address your body's muscular tension and issues.

You want to begin above your eyebrows. Position your hands as if you are about to type something and tap your fingertips along the ridge of your brow, around your skull, down to the base of your skull. Now that you are at the base of your skull, tap the muscles of your neck, moving down and along your shoulders. Keep your hands on the same sides, so that your right hand is tapping your right shoulder, and your left hand is tapping your left shoulder. You may feel a bit like a T-Rex as your mobility becomes limited. Don't strain yourself; stop when your hands go as far as they can reach.

Now, you want to switch hands to opposite sides of the body. Begin to tap the backs of your shoulders as far as you can reach down your back. Tap down the back of your arm, around the wrist, and back up the front of your arm, then down your hand. Return to the front of your shoulder. Be sure to do this to both arms.

You can switch from tapping to chopping with the edge of your hands when you reach your chest and torso. Once you reach your stomach, start tapping with your fingertips again. Continue this all the way down your thighs and calves. You can use chopping on the tops of your thighs. Loop around to the backs of your thighs and try to use a chopping motion on your buttocks. Also be sure to get the sides of your hips, as a lot of tension and emotional pain is stored there.

Conclude the massage with a nice foot massage. Sit down and take one of your feet on your lap. Tap the top and then the bottom of your foot. Switch to the other foot.

Ideally, you want to hit as much of your body as you can. Using tapping and chopping, you are stimulating energy flow and tension release. You should feel much better after having done a full-body Swedish massage.

Shiatsu

Shiatsu comes from Japan. The word itself means "finger pressure" in Japanese. This aptly describes how shiatsu incorporates pressure from the fingers into a form of massage that is meant to relieve muscles tension and bring about wellness as well as total relaxation. Receiving a shiatsu massage is a very pleasurable experience, but you can perform shiatsu on yourself for many of the same deep relaxation effects.

One shiatsu move is to get energy flowing and self-love abounding. Rub your chest up and down to get your heart energy flowing throughout your body. You will increase your self-love and self-awareness this way.

You can also promote relaxation by taking your foot between both of your hands. Dig both your thumbs into the fleshy part of your sole under your toes, as deeply as you can without pain. Begin to rub and press this area without moving your thumbs. You will love the release that this brings tired, achy feet.

Rub up and down your thigh with your thumbs to improve emotional health and memory. Try to clear your mind and really focus as you do this. You will notice your memory circuits start to reform and you can recall things that you haven't before.

You can also reach around to hit your back. Press your thumbs into either side of your spine on your lower or mid back, wherever you are experiencing pain. Begin to dig into your back (not painfully!) with your thumbs. The pressure will help clear away blockages and muscle pain.

Knot your hands into fists and use your knuckles to rub your scalp in a back and forth motion. This pressure will help relieve anxiety and depression. It will also clear your head, making concentration easier. You can further improve concentration by pinching the bridge of your nose between your thumb and index finger and holding for a few seconds.

Also for concentration, you can rub under your eyes using your inner four fingers. Bear down just above the cheekbone and press downward. Ease up, then repeat. This move will improve your clarity of mind and your ability to focus.

Another great shiatsu move is to stretch your fingers. Grab each one of your fingers with the opposite hand and gently pull. Your knuckle may pop; this is OK, as it is just releasing gas pressure built up in your finger joints. The stretch will feel good and will help ease any aches you experience in your overworked hands. Interlacing your fingers and pushing them out, then flexing them back in, and pushing out again will both relieve hand tension and improve circulation in your hands. Blood often gets cut off in your hands because of shoulder tension and shoulder muscle knots impeding blood flow, so you can really improve your circulation by flexing your hands. This helps with Carpel tunnel, soreness, stiff fingers, and other such hand issues.

Overall energy flow makes your entire body feel better. You will have a clearer mind, better health, and less stress. You will also be able to clear aches from energy blockages in many areas of the body. You can improve overall energy flow by simply applying a shiatsu move to your shin. Take your leg between both of your hands. Using your four inner fingers of both hands, press onto the sides of your shin, just under your knee. Hold the pressure for a few minutes, then release. You can repeat this a few times before switching to the other leg.

Vitality, or the will to live and the energy to function, comes with a simple move where you hold the fleshy part between your thumb and index finger between the thumb and index finger of your other hand. Apply pressure here for a few seconds, then ease up. Repeat then switch to the other hand. You will notice that depression melts away and you have renewed vigor and vitality when you use this move.

If you are struggling with your emotions and interpersonal relationships, you can help ease your emotional pain by applying pressure to the area above the base of your neck. Fold your hands over the back of your head in a butterfly position. Using your thumbs and inner four fingers, rub into your scalp.

For friendship and improving your social skills, you can hold your ear in the V between your index and middle fingers. Use the inside of your index finger to hit the upper rim of your ear. This will help you relax and perform better in social situations, especially if you suffer from loneliness, shyness, and social anxiety.

Shiatsu is a very varied and diverse form of massage. It has moves to address literally every issue that you may experience in life, from emotional issues to physical ones. Do some research on shiatsu and learn other movements and techniques to address your specific issues. One great resource is the following website:

http://www.ba-bamail.com/content.aspx?emailid=1937

Deep Tissue

Deep tissue massage is aimed at reaching the deep tissues of the body. You will often feel very sore after a deep tissue massage because it reaches areas of your body that probably have not been directly stimulated in a while, if ever. Usually deep tissue massage is only possible with a massage therapist. There are a few moves that you can use yourself to get deep-seated aches and pains, but usually you need to see someone professional to attain this type of massage. A thorough knowledge of musculature and anatomy is required for proper deep tissue massage, since this massage targets specific muscles and works them in groups.

The simple tennis ball massages that I covered in Chapter 2 are actually forms of deep tissue massage that you can perform upon yourself. Using any sort of instrument, such as a ball or the blunt end of a pen or screwdriver, will work to reach deep into your tissues. This is why you must be careful when using this form of massage, as it can bruise you quite deeply and painfully if you are not careful.

Using a tool to dig deeper into your tissues is also a way to give yourself a deep tissue massage. Focus on the areas that hurt you the most and rub them vigorously with the blunt end of an object or a roller tool.

When you perform deep tissue massage on yourself with your hands, you want to use all of your fingers to apply the appropriate pressure. You also want to use long, deep strokes with your hands. Your hands should flow, not delivery choppy movements. You can rub your arms, legs, and even shoulders with sweeping motions. Use harder pressure than you normally would and incorporate all five of your fingers in the massage.

Reflexology

This is a type of massage that believes that there are points in the hands, feet, and head that correspond to every part of the body. You can use a reflexology map to find the points on your feet, hands, and head. Apply pressure or heat to these points to bring about relief in the corresponding body part.

Reflexology is a bit complex. However, you can learn some basics here. Following a reflexology foot chart, you can find points corresponding to specific ailments or pains that you may have. For instance, if you suffer from a kidney infection or kidney stones, you would want to locate Spot 22 on a foot chart and press on it, in the very center of the sole of the foot. Just apply pressure to the area, not enough to bruise you but enough to feel it. If you suffer from a head injury or headaches, try pressing on the tips of your big toes. Similarly, you can press on the tip of your middle finger for sinus relief when you are plugged up from a bad cold or allergies. Hold down the reflex point for thirty seconds before releasing it.

Sometimes, you may not know exactly what is wrong. You just know that you don't feel one hundred percent well. You can use reflexology in this case still. Sit very still on a chair and close your eyes. Using a cream or lotion, begin rubbing your body so that you become connected with yourself and in tune with your feelings. Then begin to meditate on your body, letting your body tell you where you are misaligned. Press any spots that seem to call to you or that correspond with organs and organ

systems that you believe are misaligned.

Chapter 2: Some Simple Massages

Before we delve into more complicated massage techniques, I will show you some very simple massages that you can perform at home, in the office, in the car, or in the shower. These massages are easy and provide you with fast relief. You can perform these on your own. Just be sure not to hurt yourself and always use a massage oil to prevent rug burn and unpleasant friction.

Feet

Take a tennis ball and roll it under the sole of your feet when your feet are sore and tired. This stimulates blood flow and breaks up energy blockages. Just be careful not to bear down too hard. It can be tempting to be rough on your feet, especially when they hurt like hell, but you don't want to injure yourself.

You can also use your hands. Simply take your foot onto your lap. First, bend it forward, then back, really stretching your toes and the arch of your foot. Now gently pull on each toe; your toes may or may not pop. Finally, start at the fleshy part of your sole and work down, rubbing the bottom of your foot with your inner fingers and the top of your foot with your thumbs. Never use too much pressure. Friction can feel really nasty on your upper feet, so be sure to lubricate your hands and feet with some type of massage oil or butter.

Another great thing is to get a massaging and vibrating foot bath tub. Usually priced at a hundred bucks or less, these machines really clean and massage your feet. Alternatively, you can soak your feet in a bathtub full of warm water and Epsom salt to ease tension in them and relax them. Then gently knead your feet and apply lotion to soften your skin. Take this time to pamper your feet, since they work so hard bearing the weight of the rest of your body all day long.

Tension Headaches

There are two easy massages that can relieve those annoying and painful tension headaches that may spring up throughout stressful days. The first is to rub your sore temples in clockwise circles with your fingertips. Then address the very base of your neck. You will feel two nobs of bone sticking out at the base of your skull. You want to fit your fingers right under those nobs and rub to dissipate stress and tension. It will release your entire neck, where tension is often stored.

The second method is to lie on your back. Hold two tennis balls on either side of your temples. Now shake your head like you are saying no, thus gently massaging each temple against the tennis ball, back and forth. Then try to tuck your chin into your throat to stretch out your neck.

Often, doing yoga can help ease tension headache pain. Yoga is almost a form of massage because it uses body movements and stretching to stimulate energy flow, relax muscles, flex tight joints, and release stiff tendons. Tai Chi is also very effective at this.

Sore Jaw

A lot of people wake up with a sore jaw in the morning after grinding their teeth in their sleep. Others have a sore jaw after clenching or grinding all day due to stress. There is a simple massage that you can use to relieve jaw soreness quite easily. First, start at the apples of your cheeks and press up under your cheekbones with your fingertips. Follow the lines of your cheekbones to your jaw. Press down your jaw to your jawline, then follow this line with your fingertips to your chin. Pull the skin of your chin down with your fingertips, stretching the skin all along your jawline.

Another method is to gently stretch your jaw open. Then gently close it. Try this again. As easily and gently as you can, gradually open your jaw again and try to shift it left and right. Don't go too far or do this too quickly, as this can hurt your jaw. Using the knuckles of your fists, gently press into your jaw bone near your ears and massage in a circular motion as you work your jaw open and closed, then left and right.

Sore Lower Back

You may suffer from lower back soreness and stiffness after sitting in an incorrect posture all day, or if you are suffering from menstrual cramps or carrying heavy loads. You can ease this pain by laying on your back with your knees bent and your feet flat on the floor. Raise your back and put two tennis balls or your fists right under your sacrum. Then lay back down and let this pressure press into the two spots on either side of your lower spine. Start raising your hips up and then lowering them again to increase the effectiveness of this massage.

Another good move is to crouch on your hands and knees. Now push your knees out behind you and assume what is called Child's pose in yoga. This pose is where your knees are straight, hip width apart, and you are supporting yourself on your hands held shoulder width apart. Kneel back, placing your buttocks on the heels of your feet, and rest your abs on the tops of your thighs as you stretch out your back. Assume Child's pose again and now arch your back like a cat. Sink your back down as you exhale, then arch it again as you inhale. Sink back with your abs on your thighs and exhale as you feel your back stretch even more. This stretch effectively eases back pain, especially in your lower back.

You can stand against an edge, such as a counter, and press it into your lower back where it hurts the most. Bend your knees to reach the right spot if you have to. Rock back and forth on your heels to release and then continue the pressure on your lower back. Make sure this doesn't hurt. Back injuries are painful and difficult to recover from.

Sore Back and Shoulders

This soreness is most common in those who spend a lot of time in front of the computer or in a slouching posture. Lay on your back, knees bent and feet spread shoulder width apart laying flat on the floor. Place some sort of foam roller or large softball under your back, between your shoulders. Now use your feet to rock yourself back and forth, letting the roller roll out the stiffness in your back.

To ease shoulder tension, try this same posture, but stand against the wall. Raise your arms above your head. Tilt your head side to side and raise up and down with your knees to work the blocks out of your shoulders. It is advisable to not attempt to rub your shoulders on your own as this tends to lead to more tension in the long run.

Forearms and Hands

Typing and other forms of manual labor can really stress the muscles and tendons in your forearms and hands. Take your forearm with your opposite hand, laying your hand out flat. Now twist your forearm back and forth so that your flat palm faces the floor and then the ceiling and then the floor again. Repeat on the other arm.

You can hit the pressure just on the top of your forearm in the furrow between your tendons, approximately an inch below the side of your elbow. Press down with your index and middle finger for a few seconds, then release. Reapply pressure, and release again. Do this a few times and you will feel relief.

Another move is to interlace your fingers. Then twist your arms so that the tips of your fingers face your sternum. Rotate them out so that tip faces away from you. This is more of a stretch than a massage, but it is very effective.

Stretching is often a great component or friend to massage. The two are doubly powerful when used together.

Sore Butt

Your butt can be sore from sitting in the same position all day long. Work it out first by doing squats. Then sit with one leg bent and the other straight. Support yourself with your arms stretched behind your back. Place a tennis ball under your butt and roll around on it, working out the tension wherever needed.

You can also ball your hands into fists and sit on them, wiggling until your fists hit the spot that is the sorest. Ease yourself up and down to alternate pressure.

Chapter 3: Acupressure and Acupuncture

One of the most fundamental aspects of self-massaging is knowing acupressure. Like reflexology, acupressure uses certain pressure points and the idea of meridians to treat corresponding parts of the body. You do not rub the area that hurts, you rub its corresponding point. Acupressure is thus very easy to use on yourself.

Acupressure believes that the entire body is tied together via energy pathways called meridians. The energy, or chi, of the body flows along these meridians. There are twelve meridians in the human body which correspond to twelve different organs. The following are the meridians along with their abbreviations.

- Heart Channel (HT)

- Small Intestine Channel (SI)

- Triple Burner Channel (TB or SJ)

- Pericardium Channel (Per or HP)

- Kidney Channel (KI)

- Bladder Channel (BL)

- Liver Channel (LV)

- Gallbladder Channel (GB)

- Lung Channel (LU)

- Large Intestine Channel (LI)

- Spleen Channel (SP)

- Stomach Channel (ST)

- Ren Mai Channel (Ren)

When a meridian becomes blocked somehow, the entire energy flow in the body is consequently disrupted and your health suffers. Meridians can become disrupted by injury, tension, emotional trauma, or illness in another area of the body that disrupts the entire body's smooth function. Once this blockage occurs, the meridian's corresponding organ often grows sick. It is believed that clearing meridians can help ease various conditions, diseases, and pain in corresponding organs, as well as the entire body overall. It can also improve your mental well-being and happiness, as you feel well mentally when your body is well.

Acupressure spots, also known as acupoints or pressure points, fall along meridians. This is why you will see a meridian abbreviation before a point on a chart. These points are also by ligaments or tendons, and never directly above blood vessels or bones. Pressure points become irritated or congested with subsequent illness or injury to their corresponding organ. Pressing on them will affect their corresponding organs and body parts. It will also help free and clear the entire meridian, leading to better overall health. For optimal health, you need to have each of your meridians flowing clearly without any sort of disruption. If a point is sore, tender, or numb, then that means that there is an energy blockage or disturbance and you need to work on that point. If a point is not sore, don't bother working on it. It doesn't need work.

It does not take a lot of pressure or effort to hit your acupressure points; in fact, you usually only need to press a point for thirty or so seconds to begin experiencing effects. Never hold down a point for longer than three minutes. Once you finish pressing on a pressure point, let it rest for at least fifteen minutes. You can return to it later or move onto other pressure points as it rests. Feeling some warmth or even tingling at the site of an acupressure point is actually a good thing as it means that you are stimulating blood flow and energy flow in an area that has previously been blocked. This means that the pressure that you are applying is doing its job and working. Never rub open wounds, tumors, bruised areas, or your throat. Also take extreme care applying pressure to any part of your body if you are prone to blood clots or are taking a blood thinning medication or bruise easily.

While you perform acupressure on yourself, you want to make sure that you keep breathing during the entire process. Breath helps move energy and add oxygen to your blood. This makes your entire body feel better and it helps you remain relaxed. It can be easy to become tense as you do acupressure on yourself because you are focused, but this tension will make acupressure less effective.

To learn how to perform acupressure properly, study an acupressure body map. There are a plethora of them online. You can also invest in a book dedicated entirely to the subject for a more thorough understanding of this art. These body maps show you where the meridians run throughout your body and where different pressure points lie. Find the points that you should hit to address certain ailments that you may have

I mention some major points that you can hit in Chapter 11, where I cover treating specific ailments with massage and acupressure.

Acupuncture

Acupuncture is the use of needles to puncture the skin in the same pressure points as acupressure in order to improve the flow of energy and break up energy blockages throughout the body. Sometimes, the needles are warmed or medicated. Other times, the simple piercing sensation is sufficient to stimulate energy change in the body. The piercing sensation also releases adrenalin and endorphins, which make you feel good. Acupuncture is best performed only by trained professionals. However, you can use some acupuncture concepts on yourself.

I strongly advise against ever piercing yourself with a needle, but you can use laser pointers, heat sources, or electricity from a device like a violet wand on pressure points in place of needles. These tools often work just as well as needles. Place the instrument over certain points that correspond to your pain or discomfort and provide the heat or shock. You will notice that the discomfort or pain will start to fade as you address pressure points more and more. You can also slide the laser point or heat source along your meridians to improve the corresponding organ's health.

Chapter 4: Releasing Muscular Tension

Half of the problems and pain that you experience is caused by built-up tension. Tension is caused by stress. Your amygdala in your brain is responsible for your fight or flight instinct. When you are stressed the amygdala tends to keep this instinct on, flooding your blood with cortisol and adrenalin. You basically live in a constant state where you feel that you are in danger and you thus hold your body in a stiff posture, poised to either fight or flee the situation. While the situation may not seem like life or death, your body treats it as such by slowing breathing and increasing muscle tension.

Holding your muscles in a tense position all of the time wears on them over time. It causes them harden into balls that disrupt your energy flow and cause you pain. The stress you experience becomes caught in these muscles and remains there, hanging out, never properly leaving the body and letting your body relax. The most common sites for muscle tension include the forehead, neck, sides of the throat, jaw, shoulders, and back. You probably will find knots in your muscles in these areas or experience soreness if you are a tense person or go through a stressful situation. Having a stressful job, traveling, and dealing with trauma are some of the most common causes of the stress that remains caught in your muscles.

It is essential to let go of this tension to feel well. Massage helps you with this. But massage is not always enough, especially if you are performing it yourself. You need to learn to release muscular tension in other ways. Learn to relax more throughout the day so that you do not build up tension. Also learn to relax your muscles at the end of the day or before a massage so that you can let go of the pent-up stress from the day.

The best way to release tension is to move your muscles in ways that force them to stretch out and release the balls of energy that they are holding onto you. Relaxation is one way to do this. Another way is performing a stretching routine. Yoga is by far the best system to achieve both relaxation and stretching. Tai Chi is another great system. Both of these systems, which hail from the East, will stretch out your muscles, calm your mind out of its fight or flight response, and increase your concentration, endurance, fitness, and flexibility. They are basically miracle exercise systems that are highly recommended for relaxing your muscles.

One of the best stretches for stress relief is from yoga. It involves standing up straight and tall. Now, step out with one leg and bend at the knee. Keep your back leg straight. Slide as deep into the stretch as you can go without hurting yourself. Some strain in your hamstring is good, but it shouldn't hurt. Sweep your arms overhead, stretching them tall toward the ceiling. This is called Proud Warrior. To add to the stretch, now sweep your arms behind your back and join your palms with your fingers facing the ceiling behind your back. Hug your hands close to your spine. This really works to open the shoulders as well as your chest.

Another great exercise is shoulder circles. This comes from calisthenics but is often used in yoga to warm up tight muscles. Hold your arms straight out, parallel to the ground, and move them in little circles. Make the circles wider as you open your shoulders and stretch your arms.

Child's pose is where you are on your knees, with your forehead planted against the ground. Stretch your arms out overhead along the floor. Really lower yourself into the stretch, letting it lengthen your back and your arms.

The butterfly stretch stretches out your thighs. Sit with your feet touching in front of you. Hold onto your feet with your hands and try to bring your forehead as close as possible to touching your feet. Follow this up with stretching your legs out in front of you and trying to touch your toes and bring your forehead to your knees.

A final great pose is known as downward facing dog. In this pose, you want to support yourself on your hands and feet with your butt pointing toward the ceiling. This pose stretches your back and your hamstring and your arms. Try to keep your heels on the ground to really stretch those hamstrings. Also bend your arms and try to get your forehead as close to the ground as possible.

Of course, practicing common stretches, such as pulling your arms across your chest, doing side splits, and trying to touch your toes, are also great stretching exercises. Any stretches that you used to do in gym class in school will work in releasing tension. Just moving your body and rolling your neck, shoulders, and feet and twisting your back counts as a stretch, which is better than nothing. You don't have to adopt a super strenuous stretching routine to start to experience the benefits from muscle tension release.

Really push yourself when you stretch, so that you feel the effort. You never want to hurt yourself, but if a stretch doesn't strain any part of your body, then it is too easy and you need to try to go deeper into it. If at first you can't perform a stretch all the way, that's OK. Just keep working at it and you will be surprised at how quickly your body gains flexibility.

You should always stretch before you perform self-massaging. You should also try to incorporate stretching into your daily routine. A nice Tai Chi or yoga routine before bed and when you wake up can do wonders for your body. Getting up from work and doing some stretches is also a great idea to break up your work day and renew your vitality. Find some DVDs or videos online and follow along, or sign up for a class. You will find that stretching will improve how well you feel and how well you handle stress.

Chapter 5: Using Massage Tools

Massage is not all about using your hands. You can effectively use various tools to help massage yourself. Tools can often do more than your hands, making them more effective. However, you can also go too far and use too much pressure, heat, or voltage when using massage tools. Always exercise caution and stop if it starts to hurt.

Lasers

A simple laser pointer can do wonders when you apply it to pressure points or trace it along meridians. While the laser may not appear to pierce your skin, its warmth and concentrated energy actually does travel into your body and cause a difference in your energy levels. Lasers are great at breaking up energy blockages and stimulating the flow of energy along meridians, thus freeing up your energy and making you feel better.

Heat

Any source of heat can provide so much relief to aching muscles. Hot packs or heat pads can be placed over sore muscles. You can use warm oil or even warm wax and rub it on areas that you are massaging. There are warming jellies, gels, and oils that create a warming sensation as you rub them on. You can also lay on a warming table or electric blanket set on a low temperature.

Cold

You can run an ice cube along your meridians to stimulate energy flow. Use a gel like Icy Hot to create a cold stimulation over sore muscles. If your muscles feel swollen and hot, you can place an ice pack or bag of frozen vegetables wrapped in a towel to prevent cold burns over the sore spot for three minutes at a time. Cold is able to dissipate inflammation in some cases and provide relief from burning, sore muscles and tension.

Rollers

There are various massage tools that employ a rolling technology. Some of these tools are electronic, such as shiatsu machines that will rub your back with a gentle electronic rolling motion while you sit in a chair, or foot bath tubs that vibrate. Others are simple mechanical tools, like wooden foot rollers that you can set under your desk to massage your feet on while you work. You can even create your own tool by finding a hard object to rub your feet, hands, or back on.

Foam Roller

A foam roller is just hard enough to apply pressure to your body, but soft enough to not injure you. You can use a foam roller to roll over various parts of your body. The baby brother to the foam roller is a rolling foam stick. You can find both online or in health stores like Gaiams. It is a must-have for self-massaging.

Feathers

Stimulating the muscles is not the only way to bring about pleasure and relaxation in massage. Often, stimulating the skin can bring about the same effects. Stimulating the skin excites the nerves, leading to better flow of energy and clearing of the meridians. It can also trigger the muscles to relax.

One great way to stimulate the skin is to use the end of a feather to tickle yourself with. You can also have fun tickling your partner with a feather. Buy a large ostrich or peacock feather for this purpose. There are also fake feathers that you can find for cheap at crafts stores.

Violet Wand

Electrical shocks can work like feathers, but they also stimulate deeper into the muscle tissue. You must use especial caution not to burn or electrocute yourself. The shocks that you administer to yourself should feel more like a tingle or tickle; they should not be overly painful. You can use any kind of electrical device that you find suitable for this purpose, but violet wands are by far the most popular because they are easy to hold and operate on your own.

Tens Unit

A Tens Unit is a medical device that uses electric pulses or shocks to stimulate nerves and help with chronic pain. Investing in such a device may be a great idea for you to look into, especially if you suffer from chronic pain.

Blunt Objects

You don't have to spend money on expensive, fancy massage tools. You can actually use lots of things from around the house. The blunt end of a pen or the blunt end of a screwdriver are instruments that you can use to stimulate pressure points or massage stubborn places. They are able to deliver deep tissue stimulation quite easily. They are often easier to use than your hands, since they can deliver more pressure while requiring less strength.

Chapter 6: Massaging the Hands

Out of all of your body parts, your hands have it the roughest. They are exposed to the elements and they must do the bulk of the tasks that you perform. They do countless things for you all day long. As a result, you probably experience frequent foot and hand aches and tiredness. Your extremities deserve a rest with a nice, relaxing massage.

So many people neglect to ever massage their hands. This is really sad, since the hands perform so many tasks throughout the day and are often tense and tired. At the end of the day, it is important to take care of your hands.

Submerging your hands in warm oil or warm water with Epsom salt, coconut oil, or lavender oil in it can help your hands feel amazing. Give them a little relaxing bath at the end of the day. Then, using a lotion or massage oil, preferably coconut oil because of its moisturizing properties, start to massage your hands.

Sadly, you must use your hands to massage your hands. Nevertheless, massaging your hands will feel amazing and relaxing. You will relish the experience. Lay your hand on a surface and begin to massage the back of your hand in circular motions with your index and middle finger on your opposite hand. Turn your hand around and perform the same massage on the inside. Now grasp the fleshy part between your thumb and index finger between your thumb and index finger with the other hand, and pinch gently. Pinch the tip of each finger. Then grasp each finger and gently pull to release tension. Pinch or chop along the outer edge, or blade, of your hand.

After a massage, it can be very nice to wrap your hands in a hot towel or a soft blanket.

Just let your hands relax for a while in this warm or soft cloth, not doing anything with them. Give them a break.

If you type or otherwise use your hands heavily throughout the day, you should take brief breaks from work to massage your hands. While the above massage is great, you often don't have time to thoroughly rub your hands. Therefore, you can easily grasp your fingers and pull back, stretching the entire hand out. You can also use your thumb and forefinger to rub sore spots on your hand in a circular, firm motion. Rolling your hand on a tennis ball or rolling meditation balls around in your palm can also work to massage and stretch your hand, giving you a much-needed break from your manual work.

I also recommend going for manicures at least once a month. Manicures help you keep your hands looking nice. They also help preserve your nail health by cleaning your nails, trimming back your cuticles, and preventing hang nails and other nail breakages through proper nail clipping and filing. The best part about manicures is that a good manicurist will always massage your hands and fingers.

To prevent wearing out your hands and increasing pain, avoid cracking your knuckles. If you feel the need to crack, simply stretch your finger backwards as far as it will comfortably go, or pull on your finger until it pops. Always combine stretching with popping.

Chapter 7: Stimulating the Skin

Skin stimulation is a critical part of massage. Many people do not believe this. But stimulating the nerve endings in your skin increases your circulation, relaxes your muscles and tissues deeper down, and promotes energy flow. You don't always need a deep tissue massage to get results. Sometimes, just lightly brushing or tickling the skin can do wonders.

It is a great idea to accompany a massage with some skin stimulation. This stimulation can simply involve lightly tickling or rubbing your skin with your fingers. It can also involve using an instrument, such as a violet wand or feather, to provide some stimulation to the skin.

Stimulate your skin over your pressure points to get the same effects as you would by giving pressure. Skin stimulation can work in place of pressure if you have an injury or a pressure point that is too sensitive to press down on. Stimulate the skin over the area or pressure point without bearing down with any pressure at all. A gentle electric current, or a warm wrap, can be applied to the pressure point to get energy unstuck and flowing again. Drip comfortably hot wax or warm oil onto pressure points as well.

You should also try tickling or electrically stimulating skin over areas where you may be experiencing numbness. Numbness is typically because of a lack of circulation or a problem in the nerve endings that caused them to deaden. If your doctor says that it is OK, you can use tickling or light electrical stimulation to help bring sensation back to the area. This will not work overnight, but it will work over time. Be careful not to use too much electricity; if an area is numb, you may not be able to tell when you are hurting yourself. Heat and cold usually have no effect on numbness, though they can help improve circulation in blocked areas of the body.

Chapter 8: Facial Massage

Many people neglect their faces altogether when they give themselves a massage. You do not realize how much tension your facial muscles do indeed carry. As you scrunch your face up in concentration, tension, irritability, laughter, or anger, you are putting stress on your facial muscles. You most likely spend most of the day holding your facial muscles in the same demanding position, which contributes to wrinkles, frown lines, worry lines, and smile lines. It also contributes to tension and slight soreness or tiredness in the face. It is quite important to address your face with a nice facial massage when you can. Give your face as much love as you do your shoulders, back, and feet, the areas that most people focus on in massage.

You don't always have to take time out of your day to do an extensive facial massage. Instead, make it an easy habit to massage your face every night when you wash it or take your makeup off if you wear makeup. As you wash your face, really take care of your skin. Use an exfoliator to remove dead skin and unclog pores. Then use a moisturizer to repair dry and dead skin. As you put on the exfoliator, gently rub it into your face in little circular motions, getting every part of your face except for the tender area around the eyes. Then gently wash the exfoliator off with a soft cloth and warm water. You can use your hands and water as well, if you want. Next, apply the moisturizer in the same loving fashion.

You can remove the moisturizer with a tissue after application if you are prone to oily skin or acne; the little bit of moisture will still help soften your skin, without clogging your pores and contributing to your skin issues. Don't make the mistake of thinking that your skin does not moisture if it is oily, as oily skin is often overcompensating for dryness.

Also, don't make the mistake of neglecting your skin if you are a man. Many men shave but don't bother to moisturize or exfoliate properly. You still need to do this even as a man. It will actually help you prevent razor burn and get a smoother shave, as well as healthier looking skin. Taking care of your face also gives you the excuse to do a full, relaxing facial massage before bed.

If you feel tension in your face throughout the day, you can stop what you are doing and perform a quick, relaxing facial massage. First, interlace your fingers so that your thumbs are free. Point your elbows to the floor and place each of your thumbs on the inside of the brow bone, just above your eye. Apply pressure. Then slide your thumbs along the brow bone, imagining tension leaving your forehead muscles as you work along. Press your thumbs into your temples once you reach them, and make small circles with your thumbs, using light pressure. Now work around your head, until you reach the back of your head. You can repeat this massage as many times as you like, until you feel totally relaxed. You will be shocked at how much tension is in your facial muscles, until you feel it all release.

It is also quite satisfying to massage your cheeks and jaw. Not as much tension is held in your cheeks as your forehead, but think about it. What moves when you smile, talk, laugh, frown, or even squint? Your forehead does, but so do your cheek muscles. Your cheek muscles follow along with every facial expression you make. They are tired and deserve a nice break with a massage. Interlace your fingers again, leaving the thumbs free, but arch your fingers over your nose. Use your thumbs to massage tiny circles along your cheekbone, just under your eye. Slide your hands lower down your nose and work along under the cheekbone. Slide down once again and work over the meat of your cheeks.

Finally, do this along your jawline. Always work from your nose outward, letting your interlaced hands stretch outward like butterfly wings. Moving inwards will only cramp your hands and make the massage more difficult than it needs to be.

Avoid just rubbing your jaw, something that many people make the mistake of doing. This can actually increase the tightness of your jaw, even if it provides you with momentary relief. You should instead work along your jawline, and apply only light pressure. Also use lots of stretching to loosen your jaw up and release tension. Do not work your jaw bones in a circle.

The ears are loaded with acupressure points. They are also very sensitive. A simple, basic earlobe rub or a gentle rub along the rim of your outer ear is often very relaxing. It is a great move to add to a sensual massage, as well. You can massage the tragus, the little flap that folds over your ear canal, as well for headache relief. Massaging your ears can be a great way to conclude a facial massage.

Another great place to pay attention is your throat. The muscles along either side of your vocal cord are often stressed and used strenuously, but they do not receive much relief or relaxation. Gently massaging down the throat muscles with your thumbs can also provide you with great tension release. The more tension you release in your body, the better you will feel.

Chapter 9: Massage for Athletes

As an athlete, you may often put strain on your muscles and tendons and even bones. You may also suffer from lactic acid buildup after a hard workout, which causes the lingering soreness in your muscles that last for days. Your risk for sports-related injuries are also rather high and you may suffer chronic pain from old injuries. Being able to stretch and massage yourself properly is very important to preventing muscle and tendon sports injuries, dissipating lingering muscle soreness, and keeping yourself ready for another day of exercise.

Massage has become a staple in the routine of professional athletes. Personal trainers, sports coaches, and massage therapists have developed forms of massage specifically helpful for the unique problems that athletes may face. If you are an athlete or just like to work out a lot, or if you are starting a new workout routine, then this chapter is for you. I will show you this special form of massage for athletes so that you can remain in your tiptop of athletic performance and physique.

Before starting these massages, you should invest in a good foam roller and foam stick. Also invest in resistance bands if you don't already have them. These things can really help you get the extra mile from your self-massaging. Also, learn a simple yoga routine or some other stretching routine that you can use before you engage in physical activity. Stretching is essential to preventing injuries and makes your massage more effective. Remember that you can use gels like Icy Hot or Vapor Rub to relieve sore muscles while performing self-massaging. You can also use hot or cold packs on sore muscles.

Arms

Wrap the resistance band around your body and take one handle in each hand. Now use the resistance band for resistance as you stretch your arms out to your sides. This will stretch your arms, shoulder, and upper back.

You can use the sides of your thumbs and bear down on the outsides of your arms, moving in downward strokes toward your hands. Then move to the tops of your arms, over your forearms. Finally, get the backs of your arms.

Using a tennis ball or foam stick, lay it on a flat surface. Then crook your elbow and rub your tricep over the ball or stick. You can take the ball or stick or roll it over your bicep with your opposite hand as well. You can use the foam stick to rub down your forearms as well.

Back and Hips

Using the foam roller, brace yourself on your arm and lay on your side. Fit the foam roller under your side and roll it back and forth. This will work out your hip and sides, easing pain while stretching out the area for maximum massage relief.

Now lie on your back. Pull yourself up enough to fit the foam roller under your middle back. Keep your knees bent and roll your body back and forth over the roller. Now, using your band, wrap it around one foot and stretch your leg up, pulling down on the band with your arms. This stretches your hamstrings while pushing your back down on the foam roller. Repeat with the other leg.

Glutes

It's time to get out your handy tennis ball again, or even use a lacrosse ball. Lay flat on the floor, with your knees bent and your feet flat. Set the tennis ball under your hip and roll your glute muscle over the ball, halting at the top of your thigh. You can even continue down lower to work out your hamstring. Now switch direction and do this the other way with your other glute muscle.

You can also use an edge, such as a ballet bar or counter edge, to place even pressure across your glutes. Be sure to alternate pressure by pressing back and forth, or rocking forward and then backward on your heels. You can also use the blunt end of a screwdriver or some other tool to target your glutes.

Legs

It can be hard to reach your legs right with a foam roller. So you can use your own upper body strength and roll a foam stick up and down your calves. Then do the same to the tops and backs of your thighs. You can also take your thumbs and press down on your thighs, pressing away from your body toward your knee in downward strokes. You can rub your calf between your inner fingertips. Be sure to also rub down your shins with long downward strokes using your thumbs.

Feet

Place your foot on top of a tennis or lacrosse ball. Start to roll the ball from your heel to the tips of your toes in an elongated circle shape. When you hit a sore spot on your foot, pause, and push down slightly with your weight as much as you can bear. Wait until the pressure is broken up, then continue rolling your foot over the ball in an elongated circle motion.

Also try this yoga pose that works as well as massage. Sit on your heels, but keep your toes on the ground so that your feet become perpendicular to the ground. This stretches your foot by flexing the arch and your toes. It is a source of awesome relief from soreness from walking or running. While in this pose, if your feet still hurt, you can stretch your shoulders by reaching behind you and rubbing the soles and tops of your feet with your thumbs.

Chapter 10: Massage on the Go

Traveling is one event that makes you need a massage more than anything. Traveling usually requires you to sit for long periods of time, sometimes in very uncomfortable seats. It also exerts a lot of stress on you as you acclimate to a new environment, deal with crowds and lines, and attempt to navigate new cities or airports. Knowing how to self-massage during travel can really make your traveling experience more enjoyable. You also don't have to fork out lots of money for a massage therapist that you do not even know in a new place, and you don't have to make time in your busy travel itinerary for a massage appointment.

How to Perform Massage on the Go

Massage on the go does not require a big production. You are not required to roll out a special massage table, lay down, and give yourself an extensive full-body massage. Rather, you can discreetly rub areas in your body that are hurting you while traveling. You can rub your thigh with one hand while in the car, for instance. You can also hit pressure points related to whatever you are currently suffering quite discreetly. No one has to know that you are massaging yourself, but if someone catches you, they will probably understand.

Often, it is helpful to bring ergonomic neck pillows and seat cushions along on long drives, plane rides, or train rides. Wear comfortable shoes that allow your feet to stay flat on the floor. Try to maintain a straight posture and don't slouch. If you fall asleep, avoid neck cricks by using a neck pillow to keep your neck and spine straight and your head up. It is also advisable to keep a reasonable temperature. Being too hot or too cold can make you sore and sleepy. Bring warm socks for long flights and a jacket. Keep the car heater down and don't blast the AC. These tips help minimize discomfort. When paired with massage, they can dramatically help your travel experience become more comfy.

Common Travel-Related Issues and How to Treat Them

Soreness from Sitting

The best way to treat soreness from sitting down is to get up and stretch when you can. Use the massages that I have mentioned in Chapter 2 for sore butt and sore lower back. Be sure to massage your thighs and your neck and temples as well.

However, if you can't get up and stretch and massage yourself with a tennis ball, you can still provide yourself with some relief while you are stuck in the seated position. One thing you can do is turn from side to side, flexing your back and giving one buttock and the other a break from sitting for a few seconds. You can also sit on your fists and work them into your sore spots. Flexing your sitting muscles will effectively stretch them and help clear blocked energy.

Jet Lag

Jet lag happens when your Circadian rhythm becomes disrupted by a time change. Acupressure is one of the best ways to relieve the symptoms of jet lag, which include confusion, irritability, insomnia, oversleeping, and hallucinations from sleep deprivation. Take the blunt end of an object, such as a pen, and rub it on the inside of your wrist bone, just a quarter inch below the fleshy part of your thumb. You can also stimulate the inside of your calf about an inch below your knee.

Pinch the ends of each of your fingers. Rub them for a few minutes. The tip of your index finger is especially crucial to breaking up stress and resetting your Circadian rhythm.

Insomnia

It can be really hard to fall asleep in an unfamiliar place. It can be even harder when you are jetlagged or hypnotized from watching the same road stretch out in front of you for hours. Bring about sleep using the techniques that I discuss in Chapter 11 under "Insomnia."

Culture Shock and Emotional Stress

Emotional duress is not uncommon when you are traveling. You may be homesick, stressed, or experiencing culture shock. You can relieve this with a simple scalp massage. Using both hands, gently cup them over your scalp and press down with the tips of your fingers. Move in ever widening circles. Use light to moderate pressure.

You can also stimulate your pressure points on your shin. Use shiatsu and press on either side of your shin bone just below your knee. This will calm you and help you feel less stressed.

Hitting the spots at the base of your neck, just where it meets your skull, is a great way to release stress almost magically. Knead this area with your thumbs, bearing down with moderate pressure.

Eyes

Your eyes can get very sore from just staring at the road for hours. Keep in mind that this can also work if you are spending most of the day reading, working on a computer, driving a truck, or otherwise using your eyes. At intervals, practicing rolling your eyes vigorously. Then look sharply from left to right and right to left. Look up and down. Roll your eyes again.

Also try visual scanning. This is where you observe the room or area around you. Take your eyes off of the computer screen or road and instead look at the scenery or something on the wall. Try to look at objects that are both near and far to switch the distance that your eye focuses on.

Glancing up from your road or screen is also sufficient to give the eyes momentary rest. You don't have to look up for long. Just offer your fellow passengers a brief glance, or glance at the scenery on the side of the road, or glance out the window of your plane or train.

Palming is a good way to block out all stimulus and give your eyes a true break for a few seconds or minutes. This is where you gently place your palms over your eyes to block your vision. Never bear down with your palms or rub your eyes with your fingers or knuckles. Many people do this for relief of pressure and soreness built up in the eyeball, but this pressure on your eyeballs is actually bad for your vision.

Chapter 11: Relieve Specific Ailments with Massage

Massage therapy understands that everything in your body is interconnected. Each organ system, each organ, each tissue, each cell is dependent on and influenced by every other system, organ, tissue, and cell in your body. Your mind and body are also connected; what goes on in your mind manifests in your body. Instead of treating your body as separate parts and addressing ailments based on their symptoms alone, massage attempts to heal ailments by treating the whole body. As you learned in the section on acupressure, different parts of the body relate to the specific organ or organ systems where problems and ailments may occur. For instance, you can address intestinal issues by applying pressure to certain points on the foot. This works because the entire body is related. Thus, massage treats your body as a whole and is able to address countless ailments and maladies, and even chronic issues, because of this approach. It may not seem like you are treating a specific ailment if you are massaging an entirely different part of your body from where the ailment is occurring, but you are.

In this section, we'll explore some really common ailments that you have probably suffered or will suffer. We will talk about how to get rid of these unpleasant ailments and heal yourself using massage. These massage techniques borrow from many different styles of massage. While they may not cure you overnight, they can relieve your ugly symptoms, help you feel better, and facilitate the healing process. Many of these massages will help medication work more effectively because your body's energy will be clear and thus able to process medication more easily and thoroughly.

Migraines and Headaches

There are many different pressure points that can relieve migraines and headaches. One of the best is to press on the spots on either side of your nose, inside your eyes. You can also press on the Third Eye Point, which is directly between both eyebrows. There is a point beside the temple, directly above the point of the ear, which can relieve throbbing headaches. A great point for getting rid of tension headaches is in the center of the neck, on either side of the spine, where the muscle indents naturally. Either side of the nose, in the dimple just under the edges of the nostrils, can be depressed at the same time to relieve migraines.

Rubbing the scalp and the temples in vigorous but gentle circular motions can relieve headaches, particularly stress headaches. You can also press down on your scalp with the heel of your hand and press backward in flowing, sweeping motions.

Stomach Aches

When you have a bad tummy ache, rubbing your belly never helps. Instead, try using the Abdominal Sorrow Point, which is directly under the ribs on either side of your belly. Depressing both sides can aid in stomach aches, gas, indigestion, ulcers, and diarrhea. There is also a point on the top of your hand, in the depression beside the bone that leads into your forefinger, just on the inside of the webbing between your thumb and index finger. In the middle of the inside of your foot, in between the big toe and the ankle, there is a spot called the Grandfather-Grandson which aids in proper digestion and the relief of nausea. Also on the foot is a spot directly in the V of the bones between your big toe and the first middle toe.

PMS and Menstrual Cramps

Feminine-related problems can be relieved by two points above the uterus. The first point, called the Sea of Energy, is just under the belly button. The Gate Origin point lies about four finger widths under the Sea of Energy in a straight line. There are also two points in the depression above and below the hipbone, next to the pubic area, on either side of the body. Pressing and massaging these points can really relieve menstrual problems.

A lower back massage with your fists or a tennis ball can also help relieve cramps and bloating. Be sure to apply pressure in the hollows in your sacrum. Apply heat, such as a heating pad, over the uterus and ovaries and the lower back.

Hitting stomach pressure points can aid with the gas, indigestion, and bloating that often accompanies menstruation.

Asthma

Press on the point in your shoulder well, between the point of your shoulder and your neck, to relieve asthma and breathing problems.

Carpel Tunnel Syndrome and Repetitive Stress Injuries

Flexing your arms outward can help with repetitive stress injuries, such as Carpel Tunnel. First join your hands together like you are about to pray. Then bend the tips of the fingers in toward your chest. Then stretch your arms out with your fingers interlaced. Bending back your fingers can also help.

Sitting down on your feet, flexing the arch of your foot, can relieve repetitive stress problems in your ankles or feet. Also hold your foot in your hand and roll it in a circle to stretch the whole foot.

Insomnia

Insomnia can be annoying and depressing. It is very possible to relieve insomnia with massage therapy. Any kind of massage is shown to help you relax, but temple massage and scalp massage helps quiet your mind. Knead the temple thirty times for optimal sleep help. Press the point under your wrist bone's point on the inside of the arm, in line with your pinky, for rapid insomnia and anxiety relief. You can also press two spots directly under the knobs of bone at the base of your skull, where it meets your neck. Pinch along your spine and shoulders to force muscles to give up their tense energy and relax. The web between the thumb and forefinger is another great spot to pinch and rub in a circular motion between your other thumb and forefinger. Finally, if you are troubled by nightmares or discomfort, pinch in a circle around the nail of your big toe.

Kidney Stones and other Kidney Problems

Kidney problems can be relieved by pressing on kidney pressure points. One major one lies in the very center of the palm, under the fleshy part of your knuckles. The area over your spleen, in the breach at the bottom of the sternum, is another crucial spot called the Upper Sea of Chi.

Incontinence

Incontinence is related to the bladder, so it is helpful to follow the bladder meridian down your back, from your neck to your hips. Hit spots along this meridian or pass over this meridian with your hand or a warm cloth in a sweeping motion.

Impotence

You can treat erectile dysfunction through stress relief massage. Also, hit a point in your back that is level with your belly button in front. Known as the Sea of Vitality, this is on the Bladder Meridian and will help with impotence.

Anxiety, Depression, and Grief

Any massage is shown to help still anxiety and dissipate depression. However, a particularly effective acupressure point is three fingers' width down from the wrist crease on the inside of the arm, under your palm. You will find a depression in the bone of your arm. This is the spot. Also use the Letting Go pressure point to release anxiety and grief. These points are on either side of your chest, just under the collarbone, about four finger widths from the point of your shoulders. Be sure to breathe very deeply as you press on these points.

Anger and Hostility

Oddly enough, the middle finger, which people use to express anger, has many pressure points that correspond to the pericardium meridian and hence relieve anger, irritability, and the exhaustion that these emotions inevitably bring. Holding the entire length of the middle finger with some pressure can help you let go of anger. Also rub the middle of your back with your knuckles or a blunt object, to encourage you to let go of your negative emotions.

Addictions

You can quiet sharp cravings and calm horrible withdrawals with stomach pressure points. A good facial and hand massage can relax you and take your mind off of your addiction. Rub the muscle that bulges out in your jaw when you chew or bite down hard. Also rub your temples, just in the hollow outside of your eyebrows, in a circular motion.

Chapter 12: Massage Your Loved One

Once you know massage techniques and memorize how to hit certain acupressure trigger points on yourself, you won't want to keep the magic to yourself. You will want to share your new massage talent with other people and bring them the pleasure and relief that you can now bring yourself. Certainly being good at massage will make you popular with friends and family alike, who want you to give them back and foot rubs. You can also please your lover better if you know how to perform sensual massage techniques upon him or her.

The following two sections provide you with some tips on how to massage other people.

Really, the same rules and applications of self-massaging apply to others. You usually want to bear down on other people with lighter pressure than you would yourself, until they request that you press down harder. Other people have different pain thresholds and may not be able to handle as much pressure as you can. Err on the side of caution by being too gentle at first and adjusting per their advice.

Also, you want to make sure to avoid massaging people with certain medical conditions. Never massage someone who has a tendency toward bruising or blood clots, or who has a blood clot. Avoid massaging people with serious injuries, as you may only worsen the injury or limit his or her healing. Never give a pregnant woman a full body or foot massage, as doing this can induce labor early. Certain trigger points are known to bring about labor quite successfully, and you do not want to trigger labor before a woman's body is naturally ready or her doctor advises induction. While the risk of contracting a blood borne disease from someone is not terribly high when massaging someone, there is still risk, so wear gloves when massaging a person with conditions like HIV, AIDS, or Hepatitis C. You can contract skin diseases, such as MRSA or fungal infections or even herpes, through skin contact, so also take precautions should someone have any sort of skin infection or condition. Finally, be careful when massaging diabetics, as diabetics can have lack of circulation in their limbs and extremities which can lead to blood clots or other problems.

Sensual Massage

For eons, massage has been a commonly used form of foreplay, of setting the mood for sex. This is because massage involves touching. But it is also a way to stimulate certain trigger points in others that can lead them to feeling sexual and open. The art of sensual massage is a great one to learn if you are trying to seduce someone. It is also a fun and loving way to spice up your love life with your current partner. Learning these delicate and sensitive sensual massage techniques can help you unlock someone's sexuality far more easily and make sex a more touching, vivid, and pleasurable experience for both parties involved.

Practice

First, as you learn sensual massage, you may want to practice the moves on your own body to perfect them. You must learn what gentle pressure feels like. A sensual massage is not supposed to be rough or hard; your touch needs to be light. Remember that sensual massage is about stimulating the sensuality in someone, not working out all of their tension knots. Therefore, practice a light touch on yourself so that you learn how to bear down just slightly, not too hard.

Setting the Mood

You always want to set the mood to put someone's mind on romance. A huge part of sensual massage is setting the mood so that the person feels relaxed and sexy. How you set the mood ultimately depends on your relationship.

You probably know what your partner likes more than I do, so go with what you know turns him or her on.

If you are not sure, however, there are always a few rather universal elements to include in a romantic setting. Dim lighting, preferably candlelight, is one such element. Another element is quiet, or soft music, perhaps classical or smooth jazz. A lot of people find musicians like Marvin Gaye are ideal for creating a more sensual mood. "Let's Get it On" is one of those iconic tracks that people associate with romance. Having a sensual scent, such as vanilla or lavender, is often a good idea, as this scent is both pleasing and relaxing. You can use Glade plug-ins, scented candles, incense sticks, or potpourri or scented wax burners to release this scent into the atmosphere. Finally, you want a very comfortable setting to perform the massage on. Cover a couch or bed in a velvet or satin sheet, preferably red which most people associate with romance and sex, to create a soft and comfortable place for your partner to lie on. It never hurts to sprinkle rose petals and set out a tray of chocolate-covered strawberries. Champagne or wine is also a great addition to any romantic setting.

Another key to setting the mood is conversation. Conversation sparks the connection that fosters romance, especially for women. Having a good conversation and really connecting with your partner over a dinner is a great way to get the mood going. While you do not have to be dirty or overtly sexual in the conversation, you do want to keep it focused on the physical. Talk about skin and touch. Mention lots of words like "feel," "touch," "lips," "skin," and "silky." Lightly touch your partner's arm and lean into him or her to put physical touch on the table and facilitate closeness. Also, provide your partner with lots of compliments and ask him or her lots of questions about him- or herself, to make him or her feel special and good. He or she will associate you with feeling cared about and will want to have sex more.

If you do serve your partner dinner before giving him or her a sensual massage, consider serving aphrodisiacs, foods which inspire romantic feelings. Asparagus, chocolate, oysters, avocado, wine, coffee, strawberries, artichokes, cherries, and pumpkin or pumpkin seeds are common aphrodisiacs that you can prepare to increase your partner's libido.

Beginning the Massage

To perform a good massage on the other person, you want to lubricate your hands and their skin with a quality oil. Not doing this can cause unpleasant friction and chafing during the massage. There are many massage oils available on the market that are meant to increase libido with warming sensations and sexy scents. You can try one of these oils, or try a simple oil from your local health food store, like almond oil or coconut oil. These natural oils glide smoothly, are good for skin, absorb into skin rather than forming a sticky film, and smell pleasant. They are also cheap, unlike expensive manufactured oils. Just make sure your partner isn't allergic to whatever oil you choose to use! Some people use petroleum jelly or baby oil, but I have found that both of these tend to stick and make a mess. They also can stain clothes.

Have your partner start by lying on his or her stomach. Focusing on the back first is usually easiest and best. It allows you to begin the massage innocently, and get friskier as you and your partner get more comfortable with the touching. You can have your partner lay on his or her back later so that you can massage the frontal region.

Massage

There are various ways to massage someone. Just remember that with sensual massage, the goal is to provide sensual and delightful touching, not hard and fierce rubbing.

First you will want to address your partner's

shoulders, using your thumbs to rotate gently

and gradually. This is known as shiatsu, a simple

Japanese massage technique. This does two

things: it releases tension, which people

commonly store in their shoulders, and it gets

you both used to the idea of touching, which can

be very helpful when you are just getting to know

someone physically for the first time. It provides

a nice opening to the rest of the massage.

Gradually travel down the person's back

to the small of his or her back. First use your

thumbs in tiny shiatsu rotations. Then, begin to

use gentle compressions with your palms. This is

where you lay your hands flat on your partner's

back and press down with easy pressure. You can

move down to your partner's butt and upper thighs. Shiatsu is often very pleasurable on the glutes, which are often sore and tense from sitting all day.

Next, begin stroking down your partner's neck to his or her inner thighs. Stroke down the back of his or her thighs, then gently dip down to his or her inner thighs. The inner thighs are an intimate and sensitive area and most people associate being touched there with sex. Don't hesitate on the inner thighs or touch the intimate genital areas, however. Instead, keep stroking down to your partner's ankles. Return to the shoulders and stroke down the sides. Some people are very ticklish on their sides, so apply just enough pressure that you are not tickling.

This is the point where you can have your partner roll over. Begin shiatsu rotations with your thumbs on the tender area just under his or her ears, down the sides of the neck, to the area under the collarbone. These areas tend to collect tension knots as well. Again, keep your touch light. From there, you can begin stroking down the front of the body. Be sure to lightly but impressionably touch the nipples, which are sensitive for both men and women. You can begin shiatsu again inside the hipbones, and especially on the tops of the thighs. Work your way down to the feet. You may return up to the chest and repeat once again if you wish.

It is often very pleasurable if you also knead your partner's feet and hands. Since we all use our feet and hands constantly throughout the day, we all tend to have tiredness and soreness collect within these extremities. Kneading them is a nice gesture that says that you care. It also will feel great to your partner.

At any point, it can be nice to add a lick or kiss. Licking your partner's nipples and gently suckling on them for a second can certainly stimulate his or her sex drive. You can also add oral sex to the end of the massage if you so choose.

Platonic Massage

Obviously, there will be many times when you have a child, parent, sibling, friend, or other platonic loved one ask you for a massage. Massaging others is not always about sensuality. It can often be more about showing that you care by helping your loved one feel better. Platonic touch also improves and strengthens the mental and emotional bonds that people share, so performing massages on others can help you get closer to them.

Often, platonic massage simply involves rubbing the shoulders or the feet. It is often best to use a massage oil when you do this and apply light pressure. What most people fail to do when they massage others is to address the tension knots in the neck, under the collarbone, or in the hands. Rubbing your loved one's neck, shoulders, and down his or her back to the very top of his or her buttocks is a nice gesture. Offer to rub someone's feet and hands after they have had a long, hard day of work.

A nice scalp and temple massage is another wonderful gesture that will make you very popular as the family or office masseuse. Start by gently tickling the scalp. Then began rubbing it in a circular motion with all five of your fingers. Reach down and gently rub the temples in a circular clockwise motion with your index and middle fingers.

Many people like to walk on each other's backs. This is not altogether bad for someone, as it helps knead tense muscles and pop vertebrae to release CO_2 buildup and pressure within them. However, it often creates a vicious cycle, where someone will continue needing their back walked on for relief. Walking on a person's back does not actually cure or fix any issues. It only provides temporary relief. It is far better to have someone see a chiropractor or massage therapist instead of walking on their back for them.

One method of massage that I have found very popular is the chopping motion. Rapidly and gently strike someone's shoulders, backs, butt, and legs with the edges of your hands. This dicing or chopping motion stimulate blood flow and is a great finale at the end of any massage.

When it comes to massaging loved ones who are sore from injuries or illness, it is best to help them gently stretch. Offer to do yoga with them, so that you both get a benefit, if their doctor approves of a yoga program. Also, make sure to defer their treatment to a professional, such as a physical therapist. You should not attempt to massage a person who has an injury, as you can make it worse.

Massaging infants can be very helpful, especially in cases of colic. Simply placing your hand lightly on a baby's sore tummy can offer him or her immense relief. You can also try to bend the baby's knees toward his or her tummy. Stroking downward on his or her belly with both of your hands can help his or her digestion flow better. You can lie a baby down with his stomach pressing into your knee to give him the light pressure that he needs to move his digestion, as well. Never push down hard on a baby's stomach or perform forms of massage such as shiatsu. Applying too much pressure can hurt or even kill a baby quite easily.

Massaging kids also calls for gentleness, though you can perform many of the same technique as on adults. A soft kneading or circular rubbing with your palm can help relieve growing pains in kids. You can also use circular temple massages to ease headaches. Many kids get jaw pain from growing teeth, so you can gently apply a circular massage to the sides of their jaws, where the jaw bone makes a circle.

When massaging elderly people, keep the same principles in mind. Elderly people often have thinner skin and more brittle bones than younger people. Be mindful of injuries, as well, and be careful not to make elderly people move their limbs too abruptly during a massage. Have elderly people stretch themselves before you perform a massage upon them, to allow them to limber up. Never perform stretching for an elderly person.

Conclusion

Self-massaging is a great way to help yourself feel better. You can relieve muscle tension, headaches, anxiety, and other issues by performing massage techniques on yourself. You can effectively help yourself release tension and heal muscle or skeletal problems with regular self-massaging applications. It is also far cheaper and easier to perform massage on yourself instead of going to a professional massage therapist or chiropractor or even physical therapist.

However, always keep in mind that professionals know what they are doing. You do not have the level of training and experience that they do. Therefore, you should leave advanced massage and muscle training up to professionals. Don't try to do advanced massage on yourself and certainly don't attempt it on others. You can easily do more harm than good if you try to be on par with experts in massage.

Nevertheless, what you can do with self-massaging is incredible. This book is geared toward helping you solve ailments, aches, and pains with self-massaging. The advice contained in this book is meant to help you provide yourself with rapid relief while on the go or while sitting at home or in the office. You can effectively get over the symptoms of stress, depression, and anxiety by performing certain massages. You can quiet tummy aches, and still heart palpitations. You can even help yourself overcome maladies such as kidney stones and gallstones by hitting pressure points sitting along the meridians of internal organs that are giving you trouble.

Best of all, massage is an art, or even a science. Practice and research will only make you better. Consider this book a stepping stone that you can use to launch yourself into the world of self-massaging. Turn to other sources and keep learning. You can really expand your knowledge of human anatomy and your understanding of your own body as well as the art of massage, in order to massage yourself in better and better ways. If you love massage enough, you should consider going to massage school and becoming a massage therapist.

In the future, you can turn back to this book for reference. Don't expect to memorize everything overnight. One read is not enough to teach you how to massage yourself. But you can continue reading, learning, and revisiting this book to remind yourself how to massage yourself.

This book also can help you massage others. While you should be cautious in massaging others, and you should not perform massages that are beyond your ability, you can certainly give your loved ones pleasure and relief from pain by massaging them. Massage can really help you bond with your loved ones. If you know how to give good massages, you will definitely become more popular. You can also use massage to enhance your seduction techniques and boost the zest of your sex life with your partner by introducing sensual massage to your relationship.

All of the benefits of self-massaging are innumerable. But knowing how to perform a massage on yourself or others is a very helpful skill to know. You will be amazed at how much you can help yourself and others once you learn this great skill.

Thank you for reading!

Other books available by K.W. Williams on Kindle, paperback and audio

Lifting The Clouds: How To Support A Loved One With Depression

Meditation 101: Beat the Stress with the Power of Your Mind